Lucky's First EEG

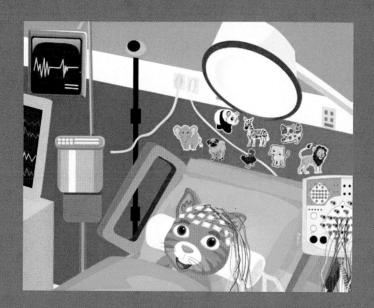

By Josie Martinez

Instagram: joseanniewrites

YouTube: Joseannie Martinez

Website: joseannie.com

Dear reader, please take into consideration that I'm no doctor. I'm only an epilepsy warrior writing from my own experience. If the events in the book don't seem to be the same for you. I'm sure there's a relatable event.

Lucky woke up feeling energized and happy. He didn't remember that he had to get an EEG today. It was going to be his first one.

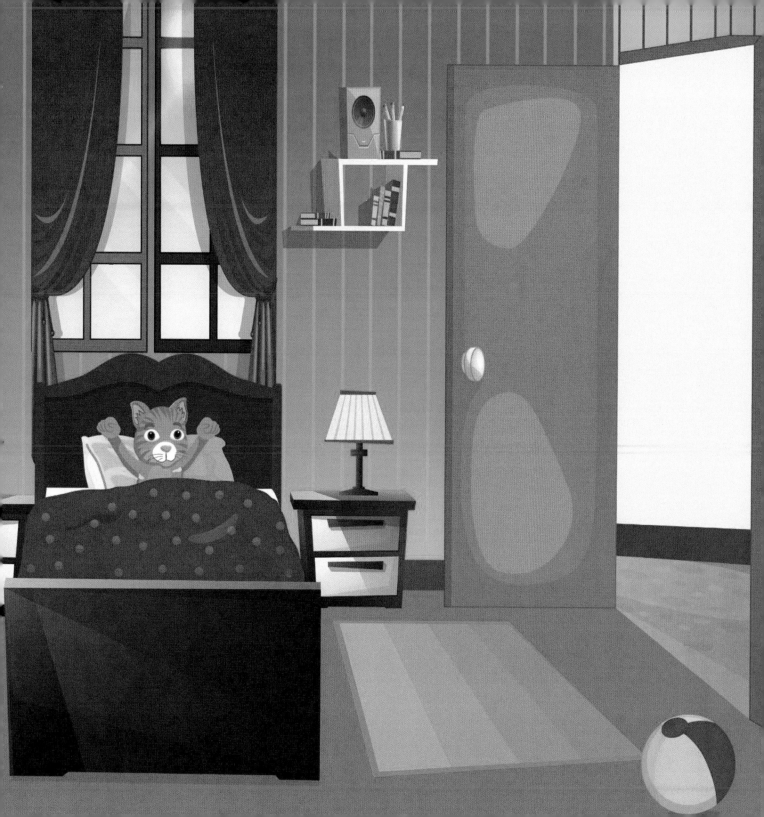

Lucky's mom came to his room to find him looking around in bed. She asked him, "Why aren't you out of bed yet, Lucky? You have to go get your EEG done today, remember?" All he could think about was the EEG. He had never had one before and was nervous about getting it done.

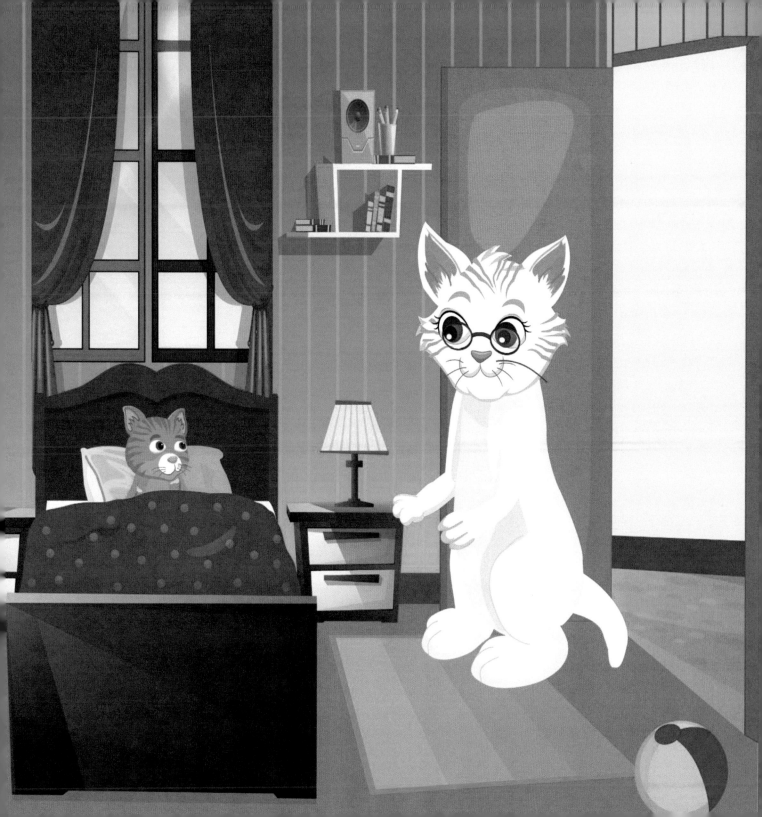

"Mom, is the EEG going to hurt?" Lucky asked as he started getting out of bed. His mom now knew what was on his mind. "It will not hurt one bit." Lucky was still nervous.

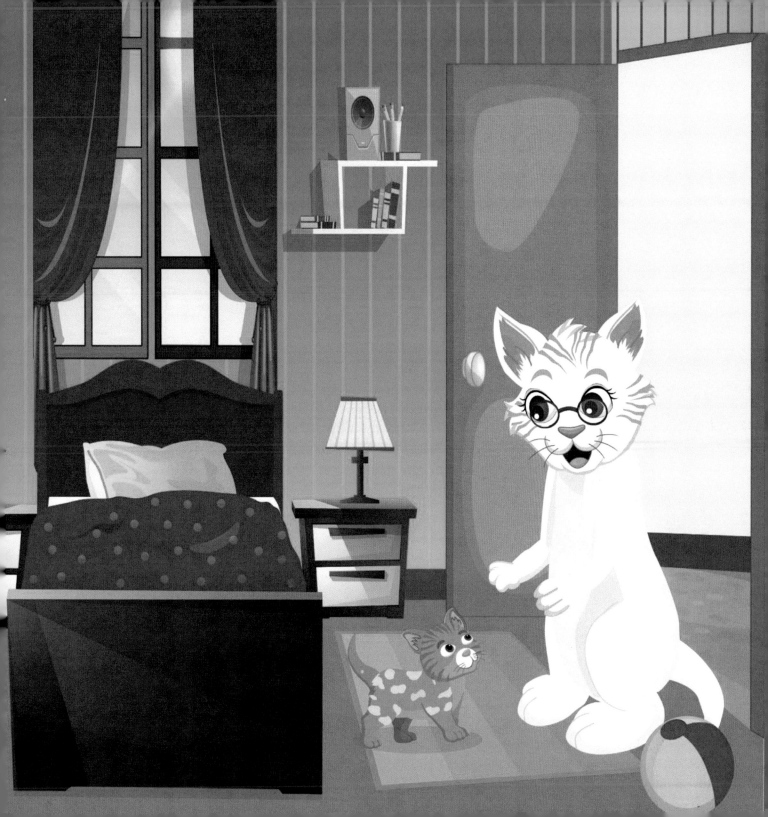

He started getting ready as his mom went to make breakfast. Lucky began to brush his teeth as he thought about his EEG.

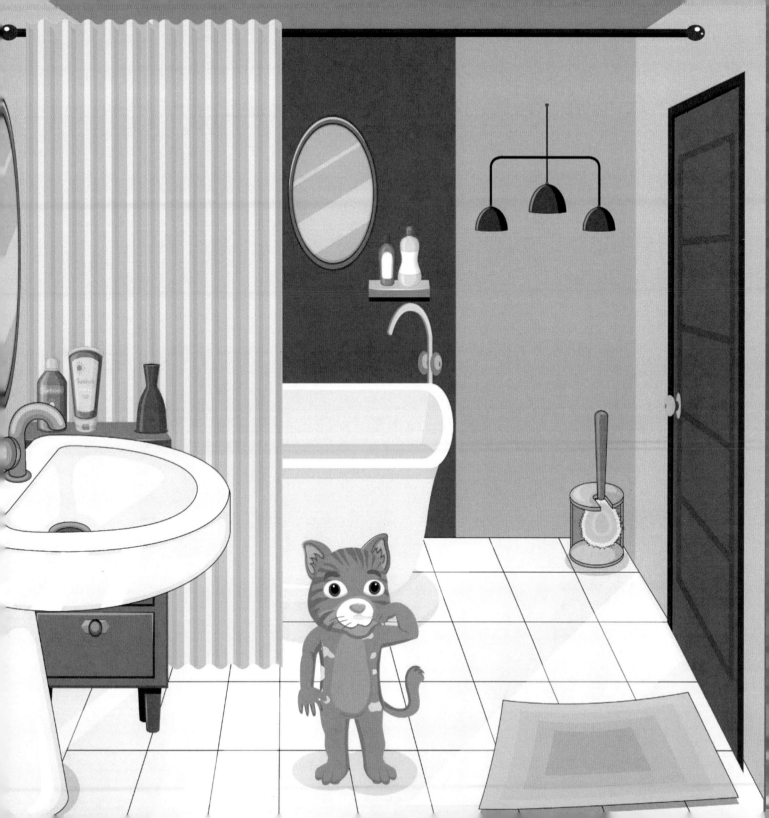

Lucky is almost ready to eat breakfast. He dries his hair well before he goes to the doctor. They said his hair had to be dry for the test.

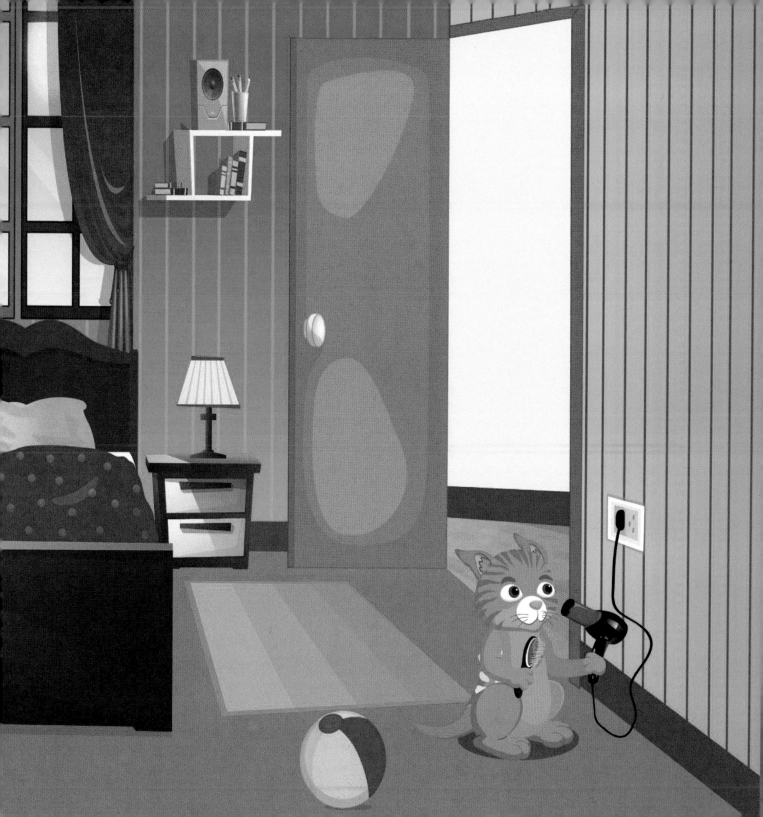

He went downstairs to have his breakfast.

Mom made sure she had everything ready before heading over there. Did she have his

medication? Check. Did she have his insurance card and ID? Check.

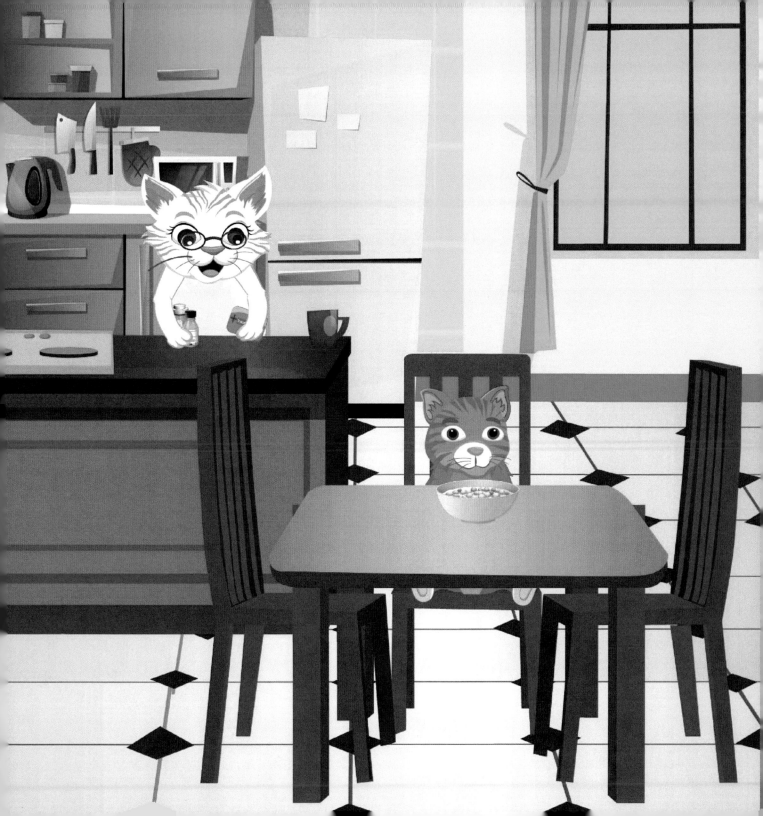

They headed out the door to make sure they made it on time. "Mom, is the test going to take a long time?" Asked Lucky as they got in the car. "I'm sure it won't, as long as you do everything they say."

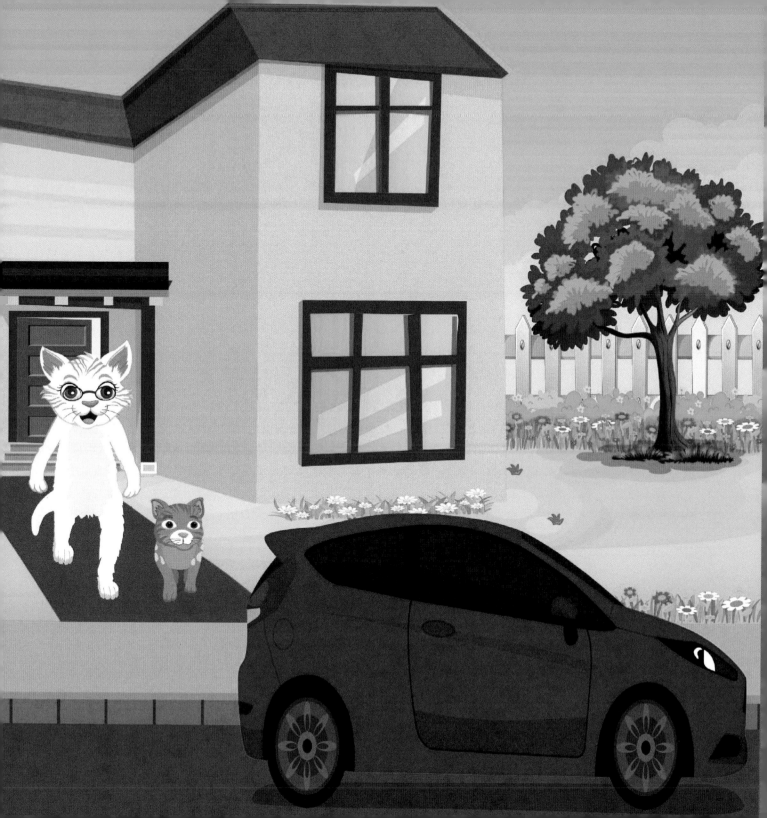

Lucky and his mom made it to the hospital right on time. The EEG tech

called Lucky and his mom in. She made sure he was ready for his test. "Do you have any questions, Lucky?" "Will this hurt, nurse?" He asked nervously. "It should not hurt one bit," she answered.

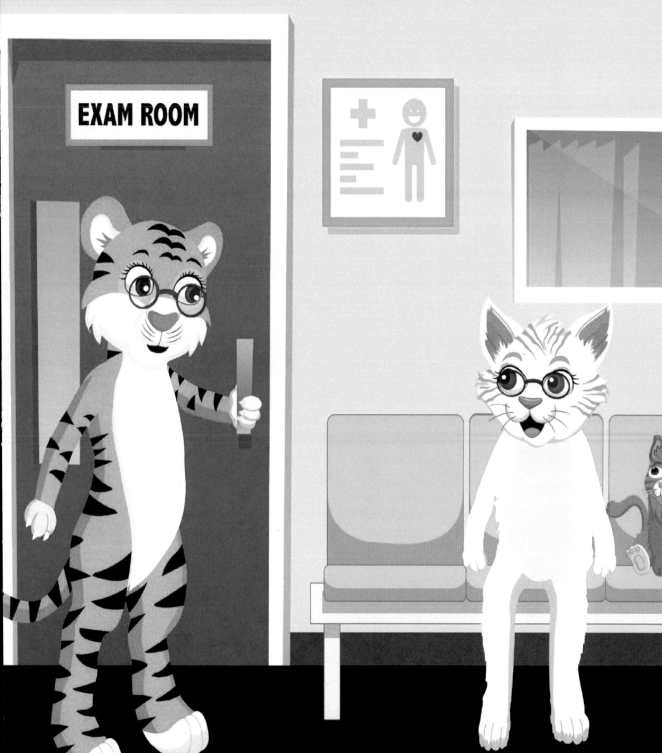

"Okay, Lucky, I will start by putting some stickers on your head." Said the EEG tech as she was about to begin the test.

"Wow, I love stickers!" said Lucky as he lay on the exam bed.

Count with me how many we put on your head.

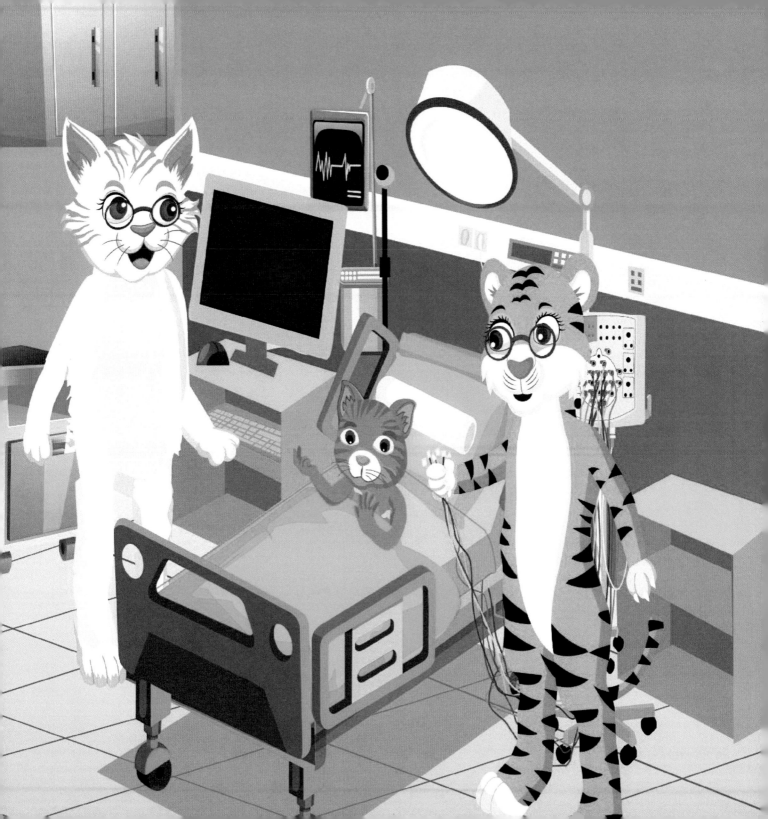

"1, 2, 3, 4, 5…" The tech started getting the stickers ready. "I'm going to use a special goo that's going to help it stick." The EEG tech started putting the stickers on his head. "Count with me again. Lucky." "1, 2, 3, 4, 5…" They said together as the tech was finishing up.

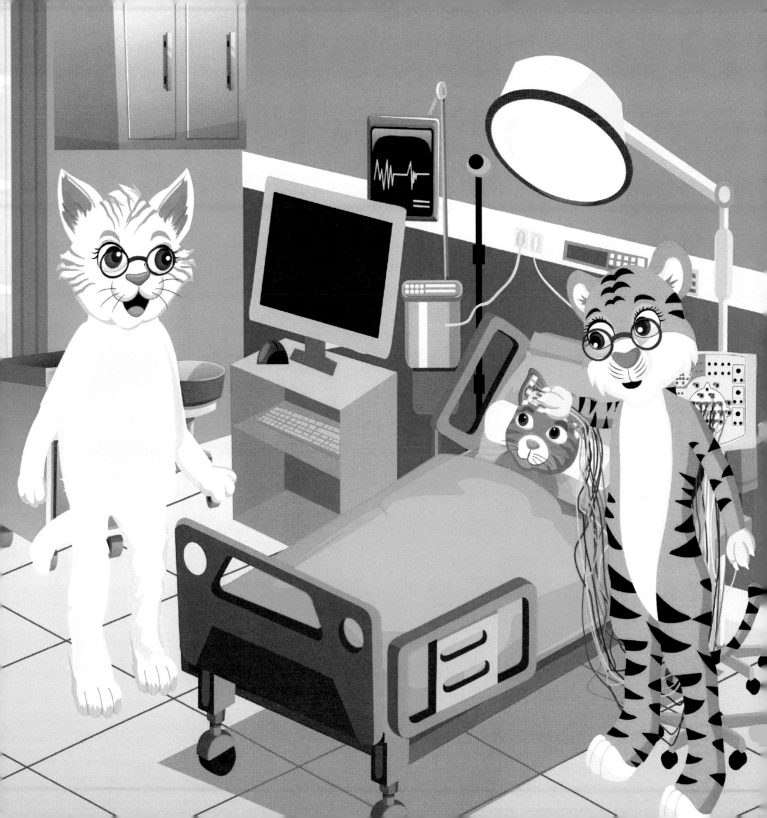

'That didn't hurt at all. It tickled.' Thought Lucky as she was done putting them on. "What do the stickers do?" He asked after all the stickers were on his head. "They check the waves of your brain," said the tech. Lucky didn't know that could be done.

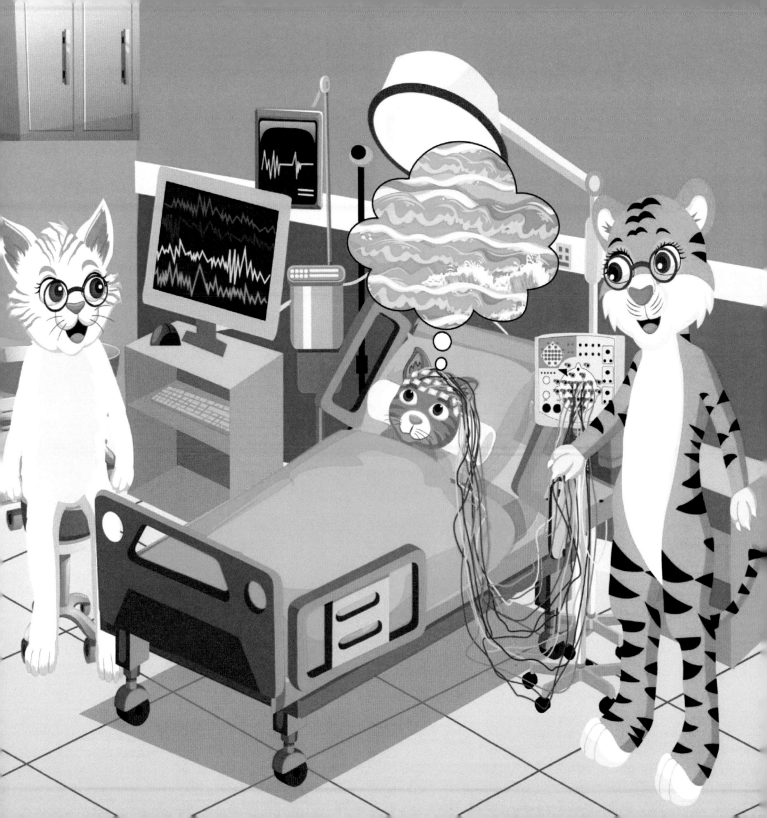

The tech told Lucky to stay still and to close his eyes. "Please take a few deep breaths." She spoke. "You can think you are at the beach looking at the waves." She said as she began the test.

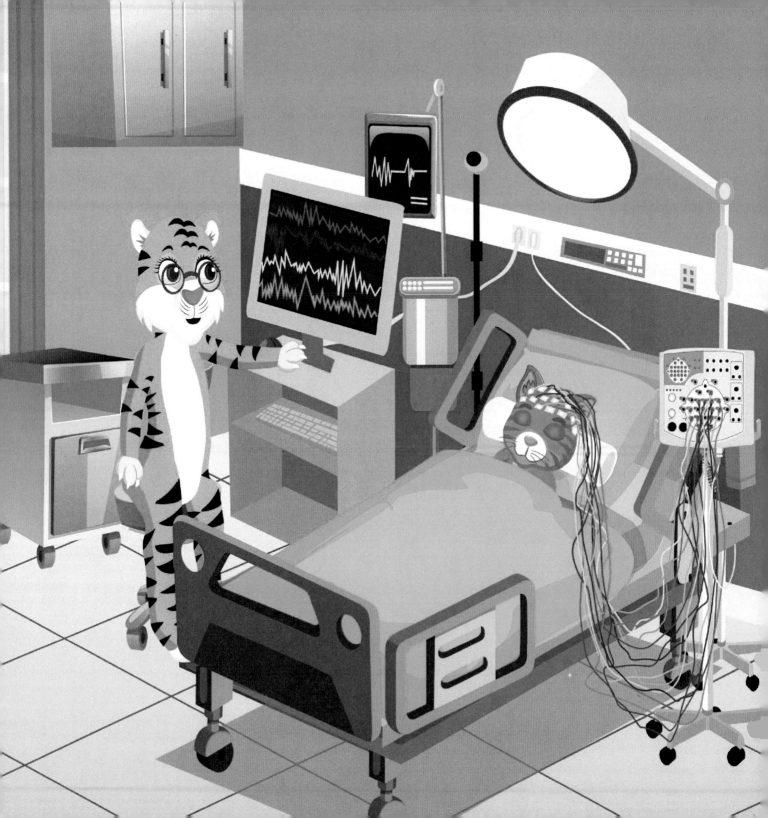

Lucky stayed very still and kept breathing in and out slowly. The tech said, "Try not to fall asleep. The test is going to take a

while." Lucky tried his best not to go to sleep, but it was tough.

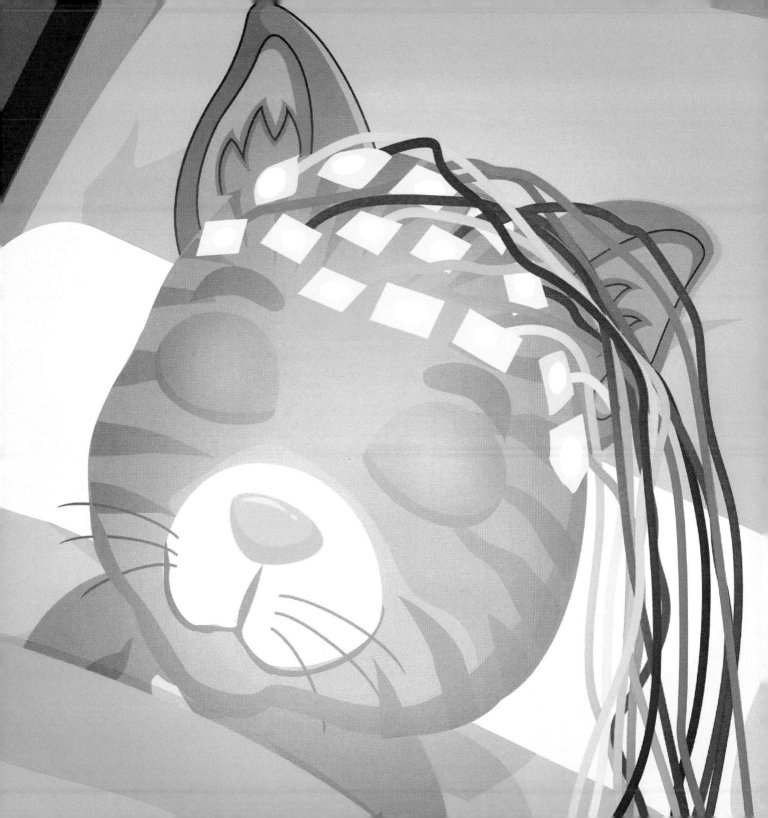

Right when Lucky started dozing off, that's when the tech woke him up. "Okay, Lucky, you can wake up now." She said as she

began to sit him up. "Is the test done already?" said Lucky, really sleepy. "Yes, we're all done, and you did great! You are such a good patient." He was so happy he did a good job.

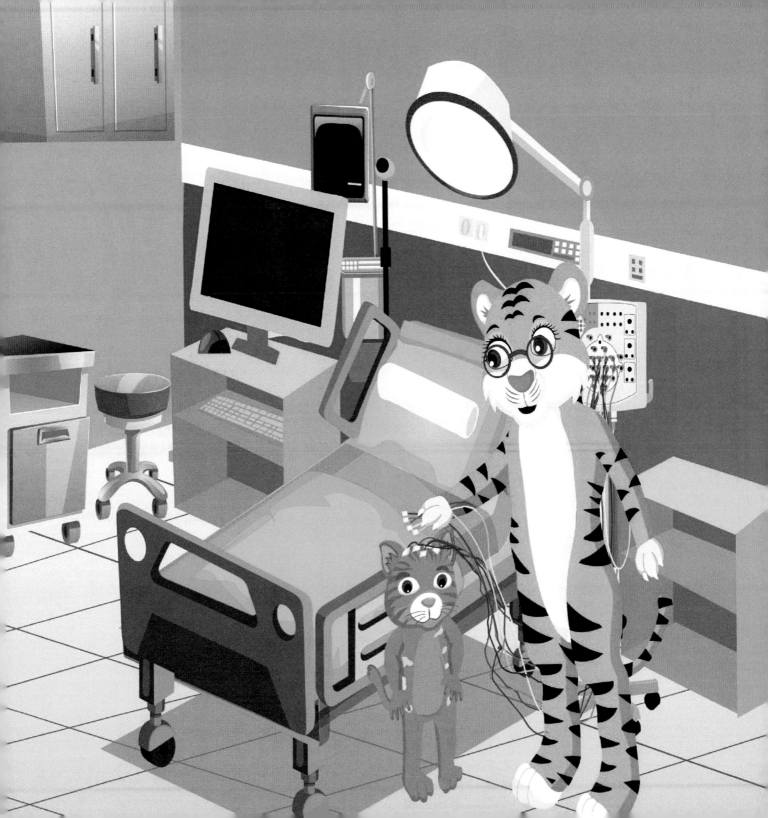

"Mom, please use a good amount of conditioner to get the goo out of his fur. The results should be ready

soon." They all walked out and headed to the waiting room. "Mom, I was nervous about the test for no reason. It was super easy." Said Lucky happily. "I told you there was nothing to worry about."

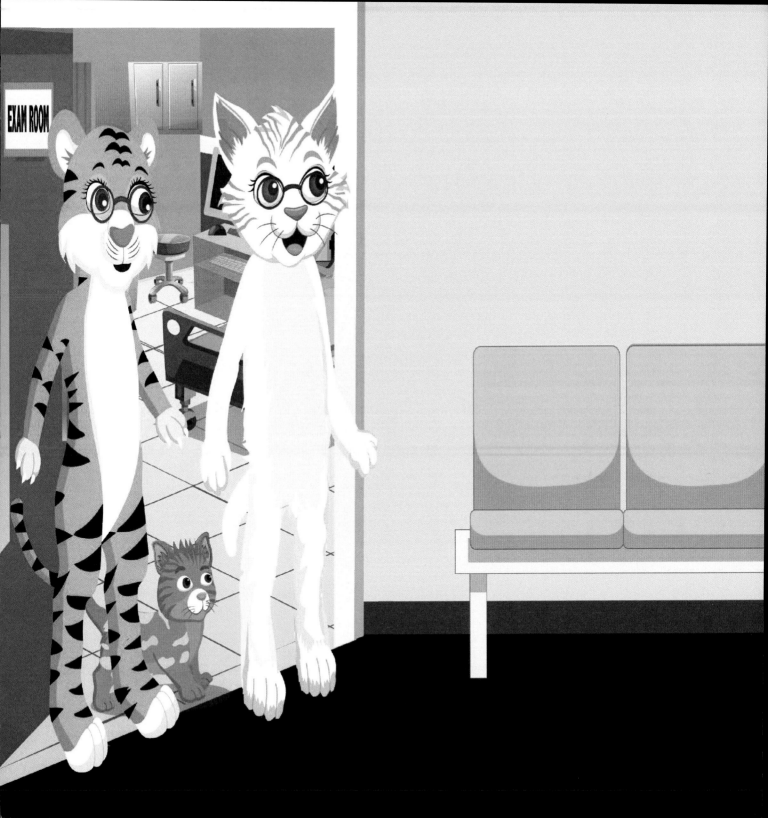

Lucky and his mom held hands as they walked out of the hospital. He was happy he got the test done and saw how easy it was. He learned so much from the tech and was glad to meet her.

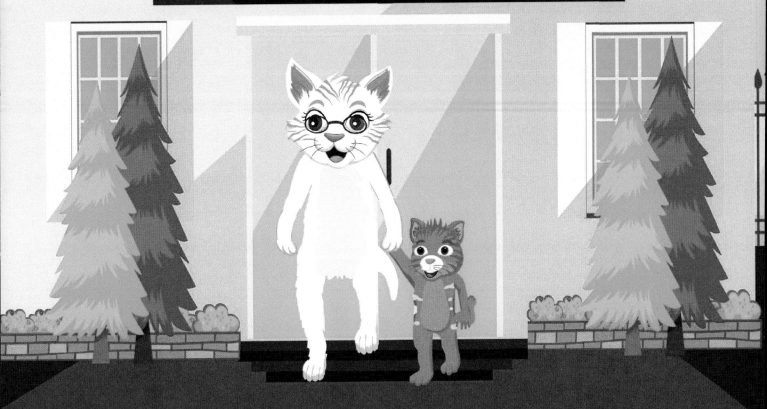

Lucky got home and told his dad how his day went. He told him about how easy the EEG is. "Dad, it even tickled when she put the stickers on my head." His dad laughed and told him how proud of him he was.

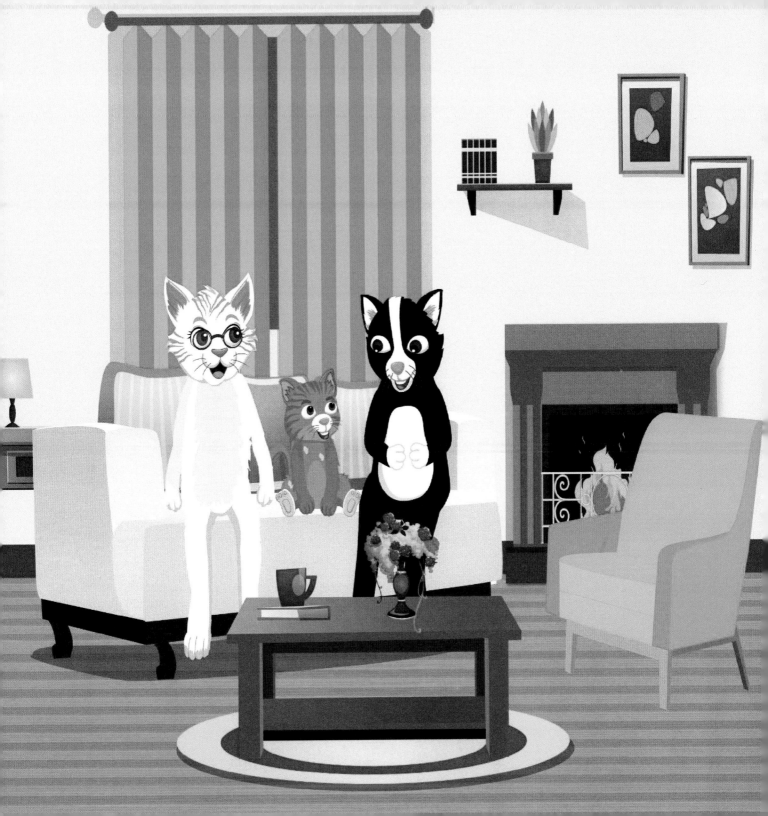

Joseannie Martinez is an epilepsy warrior who has been dealing with the condition for over ten years. She wants to help others along their journey by sharing hers. She

hopes to make as much of an impact as possible to help those with epilepsy.

Check out her other book, "Lucky Feels Fuzzy," available on Amazon and Barnes & Noble.

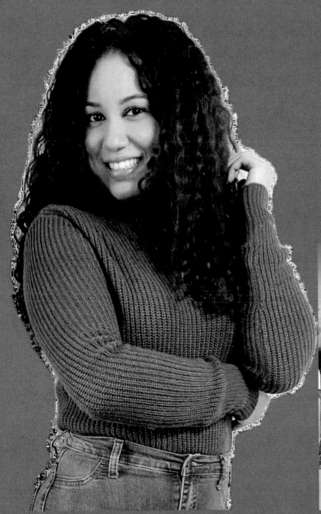

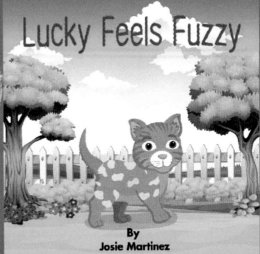

Made in the USA
Las Vegas, NV
09 December 2024

13718185R00024